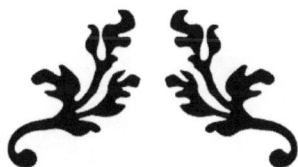

GOT SEA MOSS?

THE BEGINNER'S GUIDE TO THE ULTIMATE SUPPLEMENT

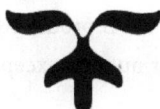

WRITTEN BY ANGELA BENTLEY-HENRY, M.ED.

Table of Contents

Dedication

I dedicate this book to my husband, Chris, and my daughters, Abriana and Aleah! Thank you for tasting, assisting, marketing, and cheering me on throughout this sea moss entrepreneurial journey.

I love you!

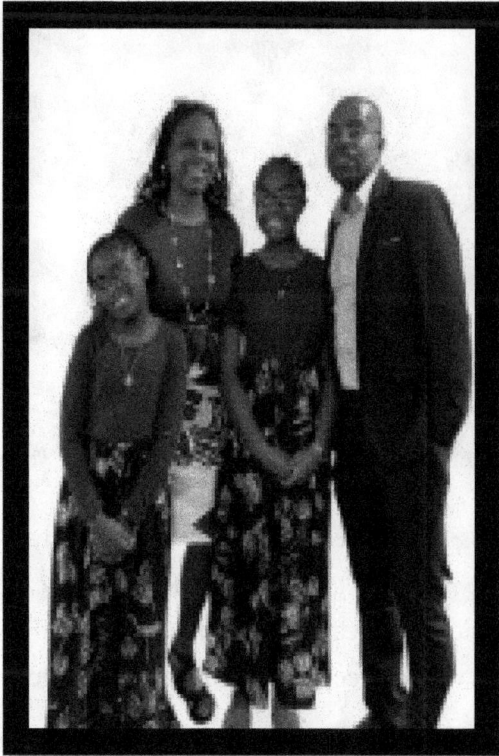

Chapter 1

What Is Sea Moss?

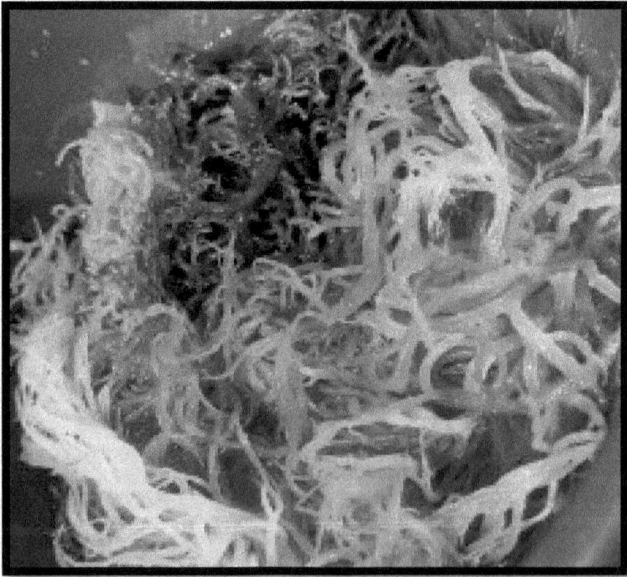

What is sea moss? That is easily the most frequently asked question I receive—and it is a darn good one. I mean, what exactly is this sea vegetable, algae-looking seaweed that holistic health doctors all over the internet (the world) keep raving about? The quick answer is that sea moss is, what I refer to as, "the ultimate supplement". It aids our body in functioning as it was designed to function.

Now, for the long answer, sea moss is a type of seaweed found in many places around the world—locations like the Atlantic Ocean, the coasts of Ireland, the Caribbean, and Southeast Asia (mostly the Philippines and Indonesia), to name a few. Most people purchase and consume their sea moss from the Caribbean Islands. As a sea moss provider, I tend to offer sea moss from Jamaica, St. Lucia, and Antigua.

Though sea moss seems like a "new discovery" to many, it has been used for centuries all over the world for its health benefits and healing properties.

There are several types of sea moss, which are usually categorized based on their color and/or place of origin. Sea moss is also distributed in many forms to include its original raw form and dried form.

Here are some common types of sea moss and their "also known as" names. This is a small list of names compared to what you can discover online or hear from word of mouth:

1. Chondrus Crispus (Irish Sea Moss)
2. Gracilaria (Jamaican Sea Moss)
3. Mastocarpus Stellatus (Carrageenan Moss or False Irish Moss)
4. Eucheuma Cottonii (Golden Sea Moss also known as Gusô)

Each type of sea moss has a slightly different nutritional profile. By nutritional profile, I mean that one type of sea moss might have a higher percentage of one type of mineral vs another type of sea moss. For example, full spectrum sea moss (which is a hybrid of a few types of sea moss) might have more calcium content than golden sea moss or vice versa.

However, even with their differences, the most important similarity is that they are all used for their potential health benefits and their nutritional additions to your diet.

With sea moss gaining in popularity, be sure to do your research to ensure you are consuming what you are being told you are consuming. Also, take time to research that the sea moss you are purchasing is being harvested (and grown) the way it is being advertised.

I will go into more detail about safety concerns later in this book.

*https://en.wikipedia.org/wiki/Mastocarpus_stellatus

*https://agri.ohio.gov/divisions/food-safety/resources/sea-moss#:~:text=Chondrus%20Crispus%20(commonly%20referred%20to,moss%20used%20in%20food%20production.

*References (types of sea moss and safety)

Chapter 2

My Sea Moss Story

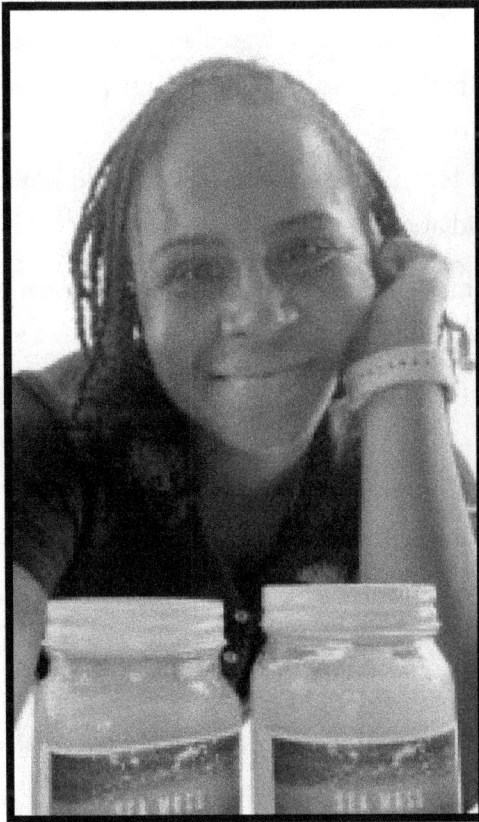

I must say, 2016 was a momentous year, unlike the previous year (2015).

In late 2015 (October, to be exact), I was diagnosed with pre-diabetes during a routine checkup and bloodwork analysis. Based on my experiences, I regarded this as a long death wish. You see, in June 2015, my grandmother lost a 20-year battle with diabetes that had been plagued with strokes, pacemakers, an inability to walk, dementia, and, in the end, kidney failure. Hearing the diagnosis of pre-diabetes lit a fire under me—a fire to be my healthiest self.

I had been no stranger to leading an active life. I grew up playing a variety of sports. I teach physical education and health, and I am a basketball and track coach. I was also fortunate enough to be a standout basketball player and played semi-professional basketball in my 20s. However, even with all my coaching, basketball experience, and teaching experiences, I still did not know as much as I thought I did about nutrition.

This frustrated me and I knew that I needed to learn how to eat and supplement healthfully.

My first dive into "let's get healthy" research was to reverse that type 2 diabetes path. That research journey led me to go vegan (whole food, plant-based) and incorporate sea moss into my life. Within 3 months of this new lifestyle, I went from a pre-diabetic A1C to a normal A1C. I also went from being overweight to ideal weight. Wow!

Some years later, I needed to dive into "let's maintain my healthy" research to reverse an abnormal heart issue that was discovered by an EKG (electrocardiogram) screening. I had slipped into unhealthy habits (eating high fat, sugary, and salty processed foods) and not being consistent with my sea moss intake and it had caught up to me.

Both research journeys led to life-changing decisions and lessons. I learned that plant-based, whole foods, regular exercise, and SEA MOSS needed to be my lifelong regimen.

Prior to those research endeavors, I had never heard of sea moss nor known anything about it. As a part of my research, I began watching testimonials on YouTube, reading anything I could find online about sea moss, and observing all the miraculous things it was doing for other people's health.

After watching Tay Sweat, a plant-based health enthusiast, speak online about the benefits he was experiencing from sea moss, I began ordering regularly from his (at that time) Tennessee-based sea moss company.

Not only did I fall in love with how great I felt, my lab numbers (bloodwork) were also excellent.

Here are just a few of the benefits I experienced after consistent usage:

- More energy
- Amazing cholesterol
- Faster recovery from intense workouts
- Better sleep
- Increased metabolism
- Better focus
- Normal A1C
- Weight loss and weight maintenance (once I reached my goal weight)

This unbelievable, healthy feeling propelled me into wanting to make sea moss available to others so that they could experience the benefits. I reached out to Tay and asked to become an affiliate of his sea moss company. I enjoyed providing sea moss to those who followed me on social media, @letshealthwithange, and to family members and friends. I did this for about a year.

Fast forward three years to the COVID quarantine/pandemic (March 2020), when everyone was looking for ways to stay as healthy as possible and to build up their immune system. Supplements and vitamins like elderberry, zinc, Vitamin C, and sea moss became extremely popular. I decided to branch out on my own and deliver sea moss to as many people as I could.

I was fortunate to be able to provide raw sea moss and gel to those looking to level up their health. I was already a certified jump rope instructor, weight management specialist, coach, plant-based nutrition author, and trainer. Providing sea moss for clients and the "LETS Health" online community was the next logical step to spreading health.

It has truly been a blessing—as you will see from the many testimonials (success stories) shared later in this book—to provide sea moss to others through my business.

Chapter 3

Success Stories

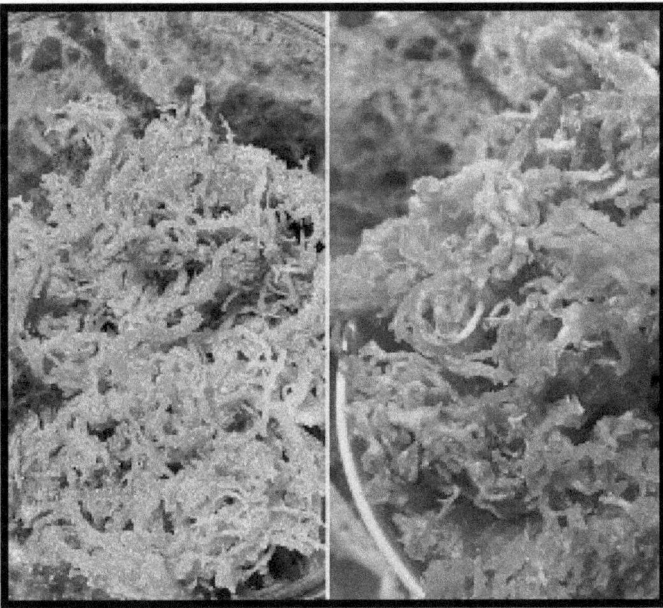

I would like to take this time to share reviews and testimonials from some individuals who have purchased sea moss from me and how it has positively impacted their health. There are so many "success stories" that I want you to hear them for yourself.

Some of the people chose to include their ages and occupations. The ages range from teenagers to 80 years old. You will read positive testimonies from people in a variety of occupational fields, such as mixed martial arts, nursing, law enforcement, those who work from home, those working in the space exploration industry, business owners, and those in the education field.

In addition to being pleasantly surprised by the benefits they have experienced, you might find yourself finally feeling hopeful for you, or a loved one, with regard to overcoming a health battle you (or they) are facing. Sometimes you just need to know that "good health" is possible to motivate yourself to make healthier choices and habits.

Personal Testimonials

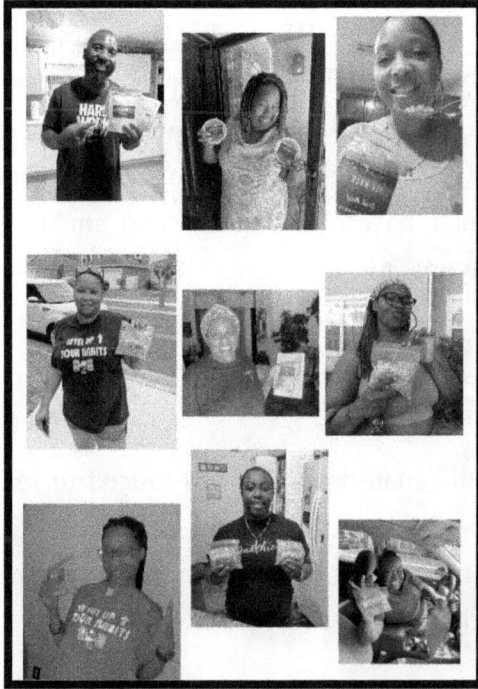

Shawn H.

I was diagnosed with elevated cholesterol and hypertension. I needed to lose weight and change my diet. My son told me about sea moss and where to purchase it. I contacted Angela and began using the sea moss.

My blood pressure is now under control, [I have] no cholesterol issues, and I lost weight. The bonus is that my skin is clear, and I have more energy.

Thanks, Angela.

Peggy W.

My name is Peggy and I have lupus along with some other illnesses that piggyback on the lupus. When I feel myself getting sluggish with no energy or no get-up-and-go, I know it's time for me to get my sea moss. When I don't have it or take it, I can feel and see the difference in my inner and outer body. When I am taking my sea moss, I am a different person. I have more energy and am not as sluggish. I recommend anyone to try Angela's sea moss. You will not be disappointed.

Mr. Williams

As an 80-year-old male who was introduced to sea moss almost three years ago. I enjoy the benefit of the vitamins, iron, and magnesium. I also enjoy the energy sea moss provides in my daily life for my health and well-being.

A Forever Loyal Customer, Mike J.

Starting [on] my sea moss journey, I was very skeptical about taking it. I had never heard of it so, of course, "fear of the unknown" kicked in, especially with everyone doing "something new" during COVID. Ange made sure she educated me on what I was taking and the health benefits [I] would [have] by adding sea moss into my daily routine. Sea moss gel has been a key part of my life now for about three years, and I take at least two servings of it a day: once in the morning before heading to work and once before my evening workouts. It does have a slightly salty taste to it, but I just chase it with my Crystal Light or orange juice. It has helped me continue to keep my immune system strong and stay healthy despite the sicknesses going around at my job or with my kids in school. I am grateful to you, Ange! Thanks again!

Patty H.

The benefits I've experienced from taking sea moss consistently for about three years are regularity (keeps my digestive system working properly) and healthier hair, as sea moss promotes hair growth. Sea moss also boosts my immune system and metabolism. Sea moss is a vital part of my diabetes management. I take it every morning in my coffee. Afterwards, I feel fueled and ready for the day!

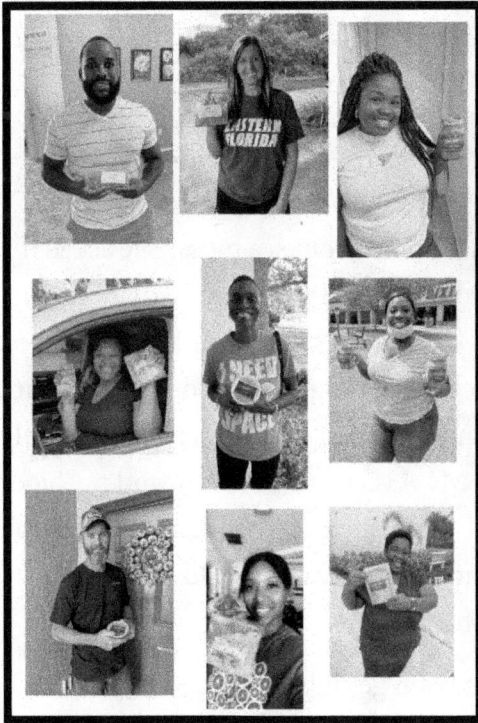

Jurace H.

Hi, my name is Jurace Henry and if you were to tell me that I'd be using sea moss gel as a daily supplement, I would've told you, "Yeah, sure." I saw one of Angela's videos on Instagram about the benefits of sea moss and decided I would try it out for myself. I found myself pushing through soreness and an exhausted body and mind a lot before trying sea moss. After a few days of using sea moss as a daily supplement, I noticed an improvement in my mood. My body was less sore, and I even had higher energy levels during workouts (I do mixed martial arts). It boosted my body in positive ways, helping me achieve my goals. She was not wrong about the benefits of sea moss, and I am so thankful that she even provided a way to purchase it as well as deliver. Her advice was a lifesaver!!!

Arlene S.

In 2020, Angela told me about sea moss. She asked if I was willing to try it, being that I was dealing with type 2 diabetes and hypertension. I'm not a fan of trying new things, but I gave it a shot. Within three months, I noticed my weight went down 30 pounds. I included walking more and watching what I was eating as well. Overall, I felt so much better. My A1C was also down, and my blood pressure was improved. I had more energy. My doctor was very pleased, and she asked me, "What are you doing?" I told her I started taking sea moss and doing Zumba.

Three years later, I am getting back into the sea moss every morning. I realize I need it as a part of my lifestyle. Thanks, LETS Health with Ange.

Terry C.

My teenage daughter and I purchase sea moss at least every other month since we started using the product. I am glad that we can purchase the gel premade. I started off taking a spoonful of it each day, but we mainly use the sea moss for our face, especially my daughter. My daughter has very sensitive skin and tends to have flare-ups more than the average person, so she uses the sea moss to help cool down her pores. She puts the sea moss on her face and waits until the sea moss dries up like a mask before rinsing it.

I will be looking to start up again with taking a spoonful of sea moss per day like I did before, because of the benefits.

Thanks for the amazing product!

Tamekia H.

Listen, if you haven't tried sea moss, you're missing out on the many benefits. Since using sea moss, I've noticed how my joint pain has disappeared. I love that I can add it to anything, like my smoothies, my yogurt, my drinks, etc., and it's tasteless. The benefits go on.

After beating breast cancer, staying on top of my nutrition has been top priority. Sea moss is a power packed supplement for me.

Do your research and get with Angela to order yours now. Love her customer service, and delivery was a breeze. Thanks, Angela.

Natasha B.

I highly recommend LETS Health with Angela! I had the pleasure of trying her sea moss, and to say it was a benefit does no justice. As a traveling, registered nurse (RN), my energy increased, my cravings decreased, my skin glowed, and my labs were remarkably improved. Ordering is easy and I received my jars in a timely manner.

5/5 ⭐

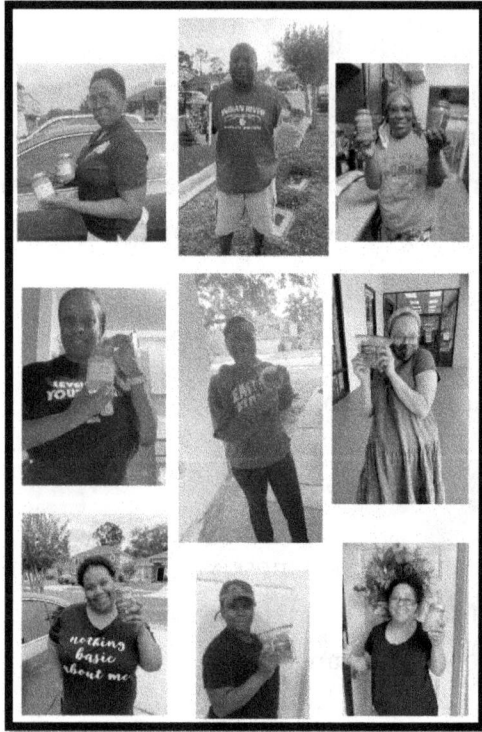

Jesse C.

I am a nurse who works overnight at times. Angela has great punctual service and consistent taste and quality of the product.

I am very active. I lift weights, play basketball, and box to stay in shape. I can tell the difference when I miss taking my sea moss gel with my energy level. Because of the benefits I've experienced, I made sea moss a part of my regimen and it's been a needed ingredient in my life.

Shylonda W.

100% recommended!! I use it in smoothies or just take it by the spoonful. Delivery is quick and always on time. I like sea moss because it supports weight loss, and it boosts my energy and metabolism. I've lost more than 50 pounds in the last year. It also provides me with the nutrients and vitamins my body needs. I love it!

Jessica K.

I purchased sea moss from Coach Henry, and I certainly noticed a difference. I added it to my morning smoothie and, man, the energy and focus I had was unreal. What I appreciated the most is there was no crash as there is with all the pre-workout drinks.

Also, there was no separate taste to the sea moss. It blended perfectly and tastelessly into the drink.

Thank you, Coach Henry. I would have never known about sea moss without you!!!

Stephanie M.

Wow! I've been taking a spoonful of sea moss for the past two weeks, and two of the obvious things I've noticed are my acne has cleared up along with having more mental clarity to start my day. I enjoy it with my tea, or I will just take a spoonful and eat it.

I have always wanted to take the natural holistic route first when it comes to my health, so when I found out about sea moss and learned more about its benefits and saw the results, I [was] more inclined to allow my body to take in and absorb the nutrients it provides. If you haven't already, try it!

Derisha B.

I love to buy sea moss from Ange because it is always fresh. I know that it's made with care. I bought sea moss to help boost my energy, and her authentic sea moss did just that. It's the real deal. I love to support her because she encourages, and she shares how sea moss has not only changed her life but helped save her life. Following her health pages on social media keeps me motivated to keep going and to stay the course of being healthy. Sea moss has so many benefits, why not try it with ANGE?! Guarantee you'll be satisfied!

Rachel D.

Ange has all the information to live your best life! She has everything from books, workout tricks, health supplements (including full-spectrum sea moss), and advice. She has you covered if you are looking to change your life!

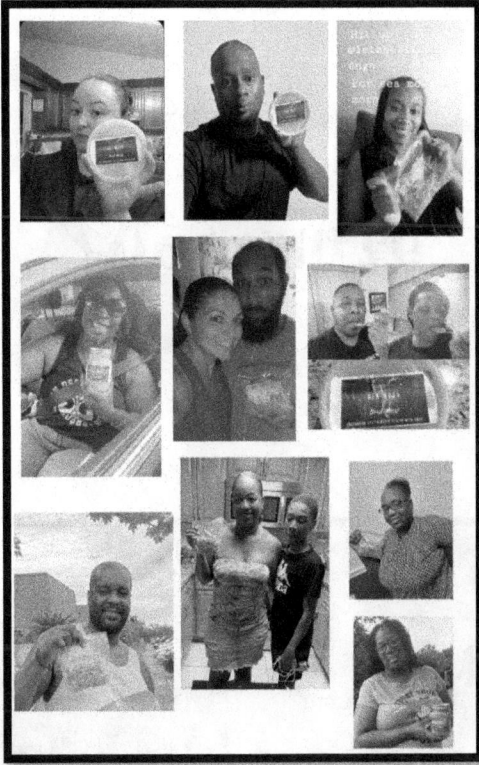

THANK YOU TO EVERYONE WHO SHARED THEIR SUCCESS STORY OR PHOTO, I APPRECIATE ALL OF YOU!

-LETS Health with Ange

Chapter 4

92 Minerals?

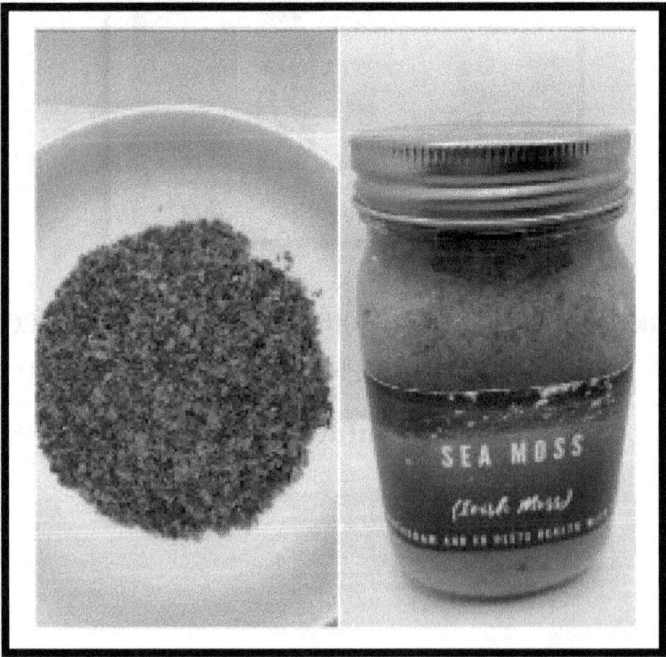

The exact number of minerals found in sea moss is often stated to be 92. Most places that advertise the selling or benefits of sea moss usually state that "sea moss contains 92 of the 102 minerals found in the human body." That statement is sometimes debated by people who do not believe in the benefits or do not believe sea moss contains that number of minerals.

I for one believe there are at least 92 minerals found in sea moss (it also contains vitamins). Those 92 minerals are made up of macro (major) minerals and trace (micro) minerals. Examples of macro-minerals include potassium, sodium, and calcium. Macro-minerals are needed by our bodies in larger amounts. Examples of micro-minerals include iron, iodine, and zinc. They are needed by our bodies in smaller amounts.

Ultimately, I do not feel that the exact number of minerals is important. What does matter is the number of lives that have positively been impacted because of sea moss consumption.

While the exact percentage of potency (of each mineral) might vary depending on the type of sea moss (and where the sea moss is from), sea moss is, as I said before, "the ultimate supplement"!

Below you will read about 10 specific (macro and micro) minerals found in sea moss and how they help the body.

- Zinc
- Sodium
- Calcium
- Magnesium
- Iodine
- Iron
- Potassium
- Manganese
- Phosphorus
- Selenium

1. Zinc: Helps the immune system by decreasing the duration of cold symptoms. It is also a key mineral for sexual health.
2. Sodium: Helps maintain the right balance of fluids in the body. Needed for muscle contractions.
3. Calcium: Great for bone and cartilage health, and great for repairing cells and tissues. Also aids in preventing blood clotting.
4. Magnesium: Plays a role in helping nerve function, muscle function, and energy production. Low magnesium levels can lead to an increased risk of high blood pressure and type 2 diabetes. Magnesium also assists with protein production.
5. Iodine: Important for our bodies to make thyroid hormones. Those hormones help control the body's metabolism.
6. Iron: Essential for making amino acids and transporting oxygen in the body.
7. Potassium: Helps to regulate blood pressure and may help reduce the risk of stroke. It is also involved in fluid balance throughout the body and muscle contractions.
8. Manganese: Supports normal nerve function and brain function; also helps to decrease the risk of stroke.
9. Phosphorus: Necessary for teeth and bone health.
10. Selenium: Might help prevent mental deterioration and improve loss of memory for those with Alzheimer's disease.

*https://medlineplus.gov/definitions/mineralsdefinitions.html

*https://www.medicinenet.com/13_essential_minerals/article.htm

*https://www.news-medical.net/health/Macrominerals-and-Trace-Minerals-in-the-

Diet.aspx#:~:text=There%20are%20two%20types%20of,cobalt%2C%20fluoride
%2C%20and%20selenium.

*References (minerals list)

Chapter 5

More Benefits

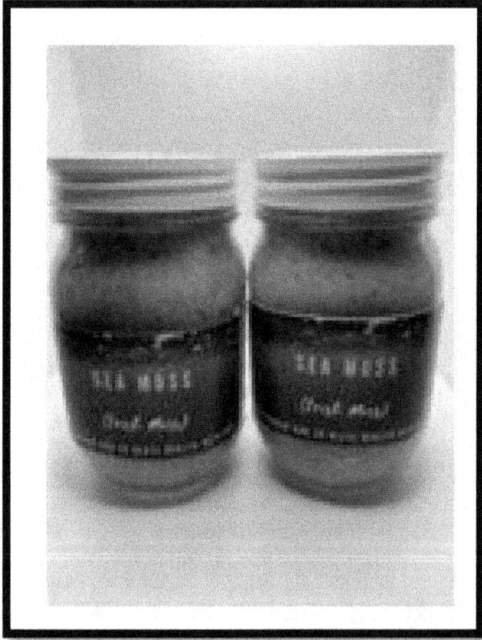

As you can see, sea moss can be a valuable addition to your diet. However, as with any dietary supplement, it is important to consult your doctor before use. It is also good practice, as with any supplement, to rotate on and off it from time to time.

This is a short list of sea moss benefits. Between my sea moss story, the personal testimonials, the list below, and the "92 Minerals?" chapter, you will get a great overview of what sea moss can do for your health.

Below I highlight some more of the benefits of sea moss:

1. Sea moss, although not a weight loss supplement, contains iodine. Iodine can help regulate the thyroid gland and help rev up metabolism. Another way sea moss (fiber) aids in weight loss is it helps promote feelings of fullness, which can prevent overeating.

2. The calcium and magnesium in sea moss can contribute to the body's ability to maintain strong bones and healthy joints. This is especially a great benefit for those who exercise often, as well as those who are older and more susceptible to injuries.

3. Sea moss is great for the prostate. Zinc is important for sexual health; it can help improve urinary function and decrease the size of an enlarged prostate.

4. The supplementing of zinc as stated before is good for sexual health. Zinc helps to improve blood flow to the genital area, which improves sexual function of the genitals and satisfaction for both women and men.

5. Sea moss is a great source of fiber. The fiber in sea moss acts as a natural prebiotic. Prebiotics help with the growth of healthy gut bacteria. A healthy gut can prevent and improve digestive issues.

6. Sea moss is great for men's health. Studies have shown low magnesium and low iron levels can affect blood circulation, which may lead to erectile dysfunction and low libido. Sea

moss consumption will help with the intake of zinc, magnesium, and iron to help combat erectile dysfunction.

7. The Vitamin C in sea moss helps strengthen the immune system and protect against common illnesses. Some people use sea moss to alleviate and shorten respiratory conditions like colds, coughs, and bronchitis.

8. Sea moss is abundant in collagen. Collagen is a protein found in our bones, skin, blood, and muscles. Collagen is important for healthy skin.

9. Due to the taurine (an amino acid) found in sea moss. Sea moss is great for muscle building and may help reduce damage and soreness to muscles caused by exercise.

10. Sea moss has anti-inflammatory properties that may help with reducing pain and inflammation of conditions like arthritis.

11. Sea moss contains magnesium, phosphate, and potassium. All are great for heart health and may help reduce high blood pressure.

12. Although this isn't a benefit necessarily, it's important to note that a 100-gram serving of sea moss contains 6 grams of protein and 49 calories.

*https://vegnews.com/vegan-guides/sea-moss-benefits

*References (benefits list)

Chapter 6

Ways to Consume

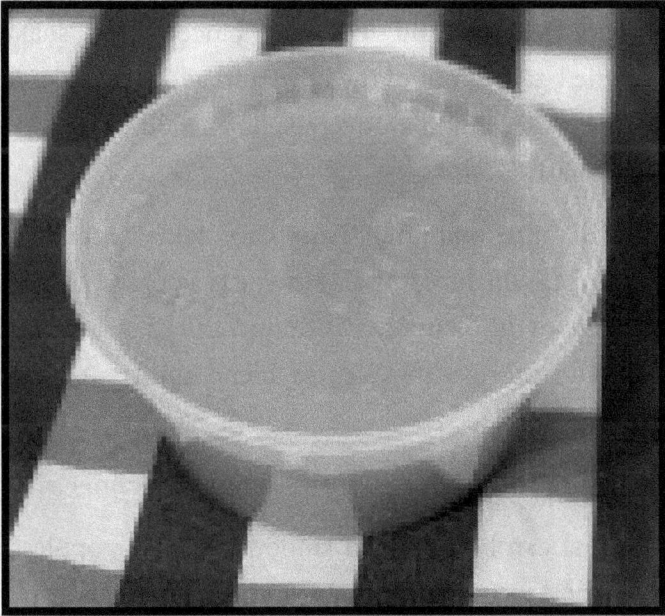

Sea moss can be consumed in many ways. I tend to rely mostly on sea moss in gel or gummy form. However, because sea moss gel must be refrigerated, sea moss as drops, powder, tablets, or even gummies is great when traveling. Those forms of sea moss are also convenient for people who live busy lifestyles and aren't home often. They can just bring the "travel-friendly" sea moss with them. How someone chooses to consume sea moss is a personal preference.

Below are common methods of handling and consuming sea moss:

1. As sea moss gel:

Start by rinsing the sea moss thoroughly to remove any debris or salt. Then place the cleaned sea moss in a bowl. Soak the sea moss in spring water or filtered water. Add enough water to cover the sea moss (and then a bit more water for when it expands).

You want to soak the sea moss for about 12-16 hours or until it becomes soft and jelly-like. Once it has soaked and softened, take it out of the bowl and add it to a blender with spring water till it's covered. Then add fresh lime juice (optional).

Blend until smooth. This can take several minutes depending on how much sea moss you are blending, the strength of the blender, and/or how thick you are making the gel. Add more water as you blend until you reach your desired consistency.

Gel must be refrigerated in an airtight container.

This gel can be added to smoothies, juices, applesauce, or even food recipes. I will share some recipes later in the book.

2. As a powder or tablet:

Sea moss is also available in powdered form or as capsules. As a powder or tablet, sea moss becomes convenient to take on the go. Powder, like gel, can be added to smoothies and teas but tends to have a "takeover" taste (depending on what you add it to). I suggest using the powder sparingly until you decide if you like it or not.

3. As a gummy or liquid:

Sea moss can also be made into gummies or liquid drops. Many tend to like these methods, as they are usually flavored and have little to no "sea taste." Also, gummies and liquid drops tend to be very convenient on the go, as they do not need to be refrigerated.

4. In recipes:

Sea moss gel mixes well with almost anything. It is great in applesauce, coffee, yogurt, smoothies, condiments /marinades, oatmeal, and even salad dressings. To be honest, the possibilities are endless. Be creative and do not be afraid to add it to different foods.

Chapter 7

Safety First

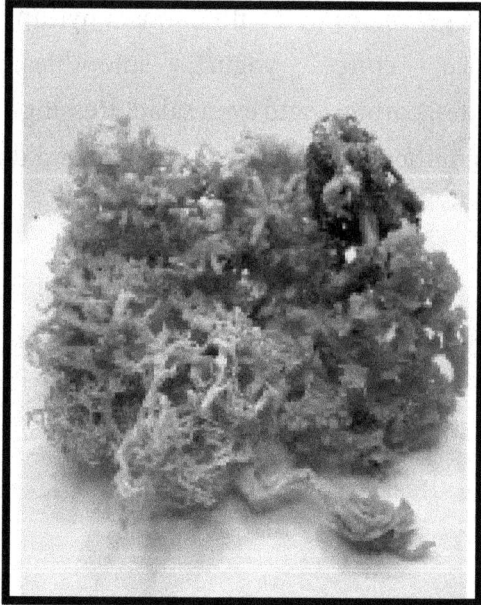

Although sea moss is generally considered safe, there are some considerations.

1. When consuming sea moss, start with lesser amounts and gradually increase your intake, as everyone's tolerance and digestion can vary.

2. Talk to your doctor before incorporating sea moss into your diet, especially if you have pre-existing health conditions, are pregnant (trying to get pregnant), a child (infants too), or if you are nursing.

3. Source your sea moss from reputable suppliers. This will ensure its quality and limit your exposure to potential contaminants.

4. Ask your supplier where and how the sea moss is grown and harvested. Sea moss can be wildcrafted or farmed (in pools or the ocean). Do not be afraid to ask suppliers and sellers questions about their sea moss.

5. Although not common, some people have allergic reactions to sea moss. Those with a shellfish or iodine allergy may not want to consume sea moss. In addition, some people might have reactions to other minerals. If you experience any adverse reactions, discontinue use, and seek medical advice immediately.

Chapter 8

Other Sea Vegetables

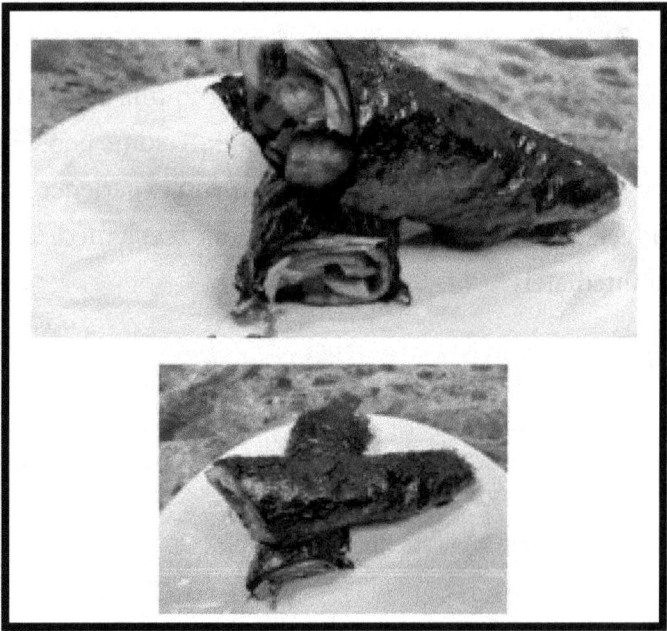

Sea moss is not the only sea vegetable available for consumption. Sea vegetables like spirulina, chlorella, nori, and even kelp are available at most local grocery stores and supplement stores. Many people cook or prepare meals using sea vegetables. Asian cuisines use a plethora of sea vegetables in their dishes that are not only delicious but pack a nutritious punch. Kelp, nori, dulse, and wakame are very popular to use in recipes as well.

Below I will dive into the nutritional benefits of five sea vegetables:

Spirulina

Spirulina is a blue green algae found in both fresh water and salt water. Spirulina has quickly become a popular supplement for its ease of use. It comes in powder form and can be added to smoothies, juices, or teas. It can also be consumed in tablet form.

Spirulina benefits:

1. May improve muscular strength and endurance by increasing the amount of time it takes before a person becomes tired or fatigued.
2. A great source of protein, especially for those following a plant-based diet. Spirulina contains about 4 grams of protein per. serving.
3. May help reduce high blood pressure.
4. May lower LDL, which is the bad cholesterol. It may also help increase HDL, which is the good cholesterol.

Bladderwrack

Bladderwrack is a type of brown seaweed or algae.

Bladderwrack benefits:

1. Bladderwrack is rich in antioxidants, fiber, calcium, and iodine.
2. May help with urinary tract infections.

3. May help with preventing tumor growth.

Chlorella

Chlorella is a green algae found in freshwater. Similar to spirulina, it is easy to absorb, and can be consumed in tablet and powder form.

Chlorella benefits:

1. May provide protection against dementia.
2. Because of its Vitamin B12 properties, it may help boost brain power. Also, if you follow a plant-based diet, B12 is a necessary supplement to your diet.
3. May help rid the body of toxins such as mercury.

Nori Seaweed

A seaweed that is commonly used in dishes that can be consumed dried or fresh.

Nori benefits:

1. Nori is a fiber rich nutrient which may help with weight loss by suppressing hunger.
2. Good for thyroid function.
3. May improve heart health.

Kelp

Kelp is a type of seaweed that is brown in color and grows in saltwater. It can be eaten raw or cooked.

Kelp benefits:

1. Great source of iodine, calcium, iron, magnesium, folate, and Vitamin A.
2. May help increase energy levels.
3. May help boost brain function.

Chapter 9

Delicious Recipes

Sea moss gel is very versatile and can be used in a variety of recipes. Whether you are making a smoothie, soup, or snack, sea moss can add flavor, texture, and nutrition to your meals. Experiment with these recipes and discover new ways to incorporate sea moss into your diet.

Smoothies

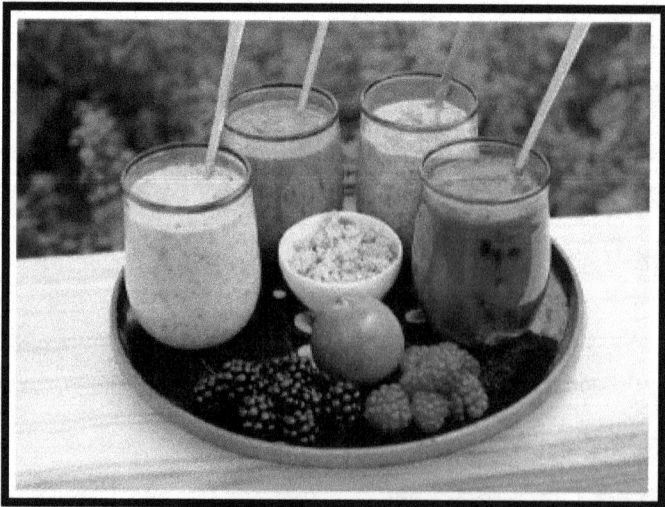

Sea moss can easily be added to smoothies. In addition to the benefits of the other ingredients in the smoothie, sea moss will add all the benefits of its vitamins and minerals.

Tropical Sea Moss Smoothie

Ingredients

- 1 cup pineapple
- 1 ripe banana (frozen)
- 1 cup plant-based milk
- 1 tablespoon sea moss gel
- 1 handful of spinach

Instructions

1. In a blender, blend 1 cup of cut pineapple, 1 banana, 1 cup of non-dairy nut milk, 1 tablespoon sea moss gel, and a handful of spinach.
2. Blend until smooth.

Caribbean Sea Moss Smoothie

Ingredients

- 1 tablespoon sea moss gel
- 1 cup coconut water
- 1 ripe mango, peeled and diced
- 1 ripe banana
- 1 cup pineapple chunks
- 1 tablespoon lime juice
- Optional: sweetener of choice (such as honey, agave nectar, or dates)

Instructions

1. In a blender, combine all the ingredients and blend until smooth and creamy.
2. Taste and add sweetener if desired.
3. Pour into glasses and serve chilled.

Berry Nutty Sea Moss Smoothie

Ingredients

- 1 tablespoon sea moss gel
- 1 cup almond milk (or any plant-based milk)
- 1 cup mixed berries (strawberries, blueberries, raspberries)
- 1 ripe banana (frozen)
- 1 tablespoon chia seeds
- 1 tablespoon nut butter (such as almond or peanut butter)

Instructions

1. In a blender, combine all the ingredients and blend until smooth and creamy.
2. Pour into glasses and serve chilled.

Getting Green Sea Moss Smoothie

Ingredients

- 1 tablespoon sea moss gel
- 1 handful of spinach
- 1 ripe banana (frozen)
- 1 cup pineapple chunks
- 1 tablespoon lemon juice

- 1 cup coconut water

Instructions

1. In a blender, combine all the ingredients and blend until smooth and creamy.
2. Pour into glasses and serve chilled.

When it comes to making enjoyable smoothies, here are some tips I've picked up along the way:

1. Feel free to customize your smoothies by adding your favorite ingredients such as flaxseeds, protein powder, or other fruits.
2. Adjust the liquid quantity to achieve your preferred consistency.
3. If you don't like a particular ingredient, do not add it, or add only a small quantity of it.

Soup

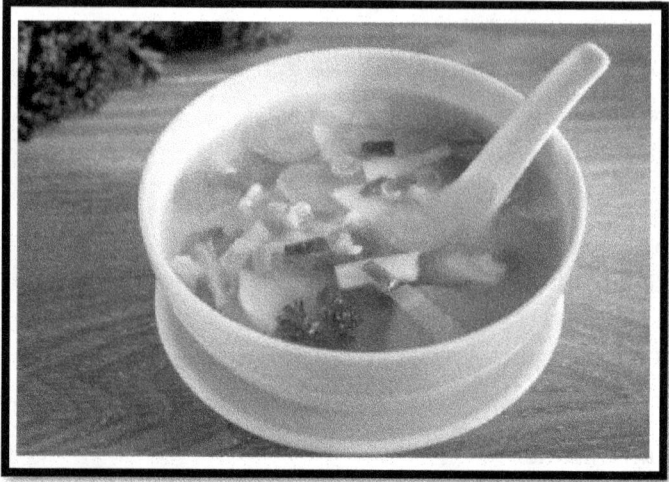

Sea moss can be added to soups and stews to create a thick and creamy texture.

Veggie Sea Moss Soup

Ingredients

- 1/2 diced onion (any type)
- 1/2 tablespoon minced garlic
- 2 diced and peeled carrots
- Vegetable broth (desired consistency)
- 2 boiled and diced potatoes (if organic, leave skin on and clean well)
- 1 can diced tomatoes (any seasoned variety will do)
- 1/2 diced bell pepper (any type)
- 2 tablespoons sea moss gel

Instructions

1. Sauté onions, garlic, bell peppers, and chopped carrots in a saucepan with 2 tablespoons vegetable broth.
2. Once the vegetables are softened, add in sea moss gel, boiled and chopped potatoes, and can of tomatoes.
3. Add in any dry seasonings of your choice.
4. Add in more vegetable broth (to desired soup consistency)
5. Simmer until vegetables are tender.

Desserts and Snacks

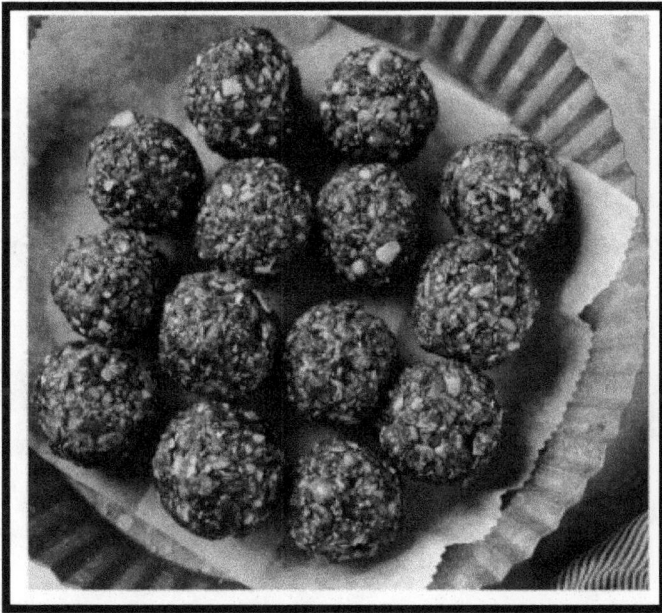

Sea moss can also be used to make tasty desserts, snacks, and condiments.

Sea Moss Chocolate Pudding

Ingredients

- 1/4 cup sea moss gel
- 1 ripe avocado, peeled and pitted
- 1/2 cup plant-based milk (almond, coconut, cashew, or oat milk)
- 1/4 cup cacao powder
- 1/4 cup maple syrup
- 1 teaspoon vanilla extract
- 1-2 Pinches of sea salt
- Optional toppings: fresh berries, chopped nuts, shredded coconut

Instructions

1. In a blender, blend the sea moss gel, avocado, cacao powder, maple syrup, plant milk and vanilla extract until smooth.
2. Pour into a glass container with a lid.
3. Chill in the fridge for a minimum of 1 hour to allow it to set before serving.

Sea Moss Energy Balls

Ingredients

- 1 tablespoon sea moss gel
- 1 cup soaked and pitted Medjool dates (about 10-12 dates)
- 1/4 cup soaked cashews or walnuts (honestly, any nut will work)
- 1 tablespoon nut butter (almond works well)

Instructions

1. Place all the ingredients in a food processor. Pulse until well combined.
2. Roll into balls using your hands.
3. Place the rolls onto parchment paper, then chill in the fridge for 30 minutes.
4. Store in zip-lock bags or an airtight container in the refrigerator.

Banana Caramel Nice Cream

Ingredients

- 2 ripe bananas (frozen)
- 1 tablespoon vanilla extract
- 1 tablespoon sea moss gel
- 2 teaspoon cinnamon
- 1 tablespoon agave nectar
- 4 Medjool dates
- Almonds (optional)

Instructions

1. First, make the caramel date sauce – combine 4 Medjool dates, sea moss gel, and agave in a blender. (set aside.)
2. Combine all other ingredients in the blender and blend. (it will be thick.)
3. Pour the nice cream into a bowl. Top with caramel date sauce.
4. Add crushed almonds on top (optional).

Dressings, Dips, and Sauces

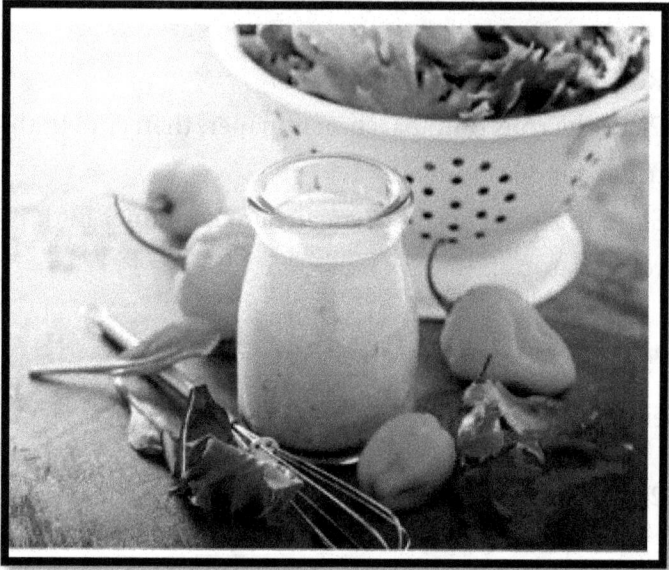

Sea moss can be used for condiments, as it makes for a great thickening agent and combines well with other ingredients.

Sea Moss 3-2-1 Salad Dressing

Ingredients

- 1 tablespoon sea moss gel
- 3 tablespoons balsamic vinegar
- 2 tablespoons pure maple syrup
- 1 teaspoon dijon mustard

Instructions

1. Using a whisk or a blender, mix the sea moss gel, balsamic vinegar, pure maple syrup, and dijon mustard until smooth.

2. Pour it into a jar or directly onto the salad.
3. Shake before serving.
4. Keep it refrigerated.

Sea Moss Guacamole

Ingredients

- 1 tablespoon sea moss gel
- 1 ripe avocado, peeled and pitted
- 1/2 finely chopped onion
- 1/2 medium-sized tomato, diced
- 2 juiced limes
- 1/2 tablespoon garlic powder
- Salt, pepper, cayenne pepper, and oregano (to taste)

Instructions

1. In a mixing bowl, mash the avocado.
2. Dice the onion and tomato. Add into mixing bowl.
3. Add the juiced lime, and dry seasonings.
4. Mix all ingredients well.
5. Cover and refrigerate for at least 30 minutes.
6. Serve chilled.

Chapter 10

Frequently Asked Questions

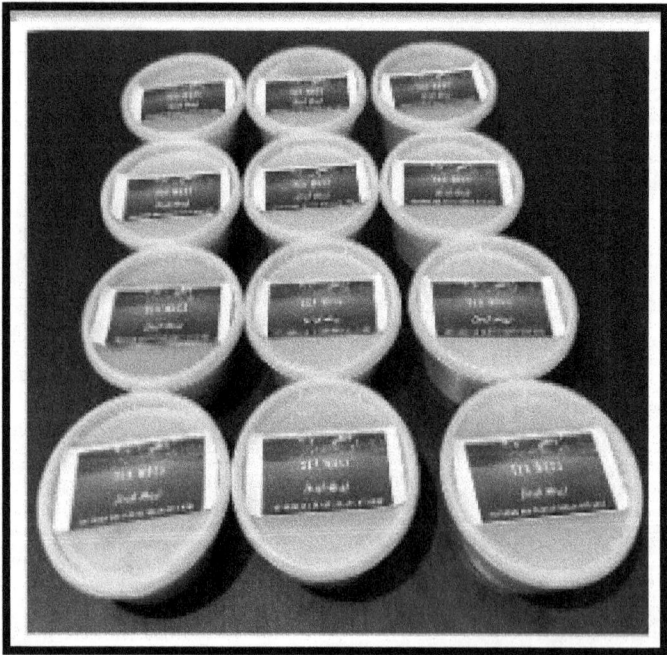

1. What is sea moss?

Sea moss is a type of seaweed that grows in various locations around the world.

2. What are the benefits of sea moss?

Sea moss is believed to have various health benefits, including supporting thyroid function, boosting the immune system, promoting digestion, supporting joint and bone health, enhancing skin health, and providing respiratory support. It is also rich in essential minerals and vitamins.

3. How do I prepare sea moss for consumption?

Rinse, soak, and blend the sea moss, then store in an airtight container. Review the "Ways to Consume" chapter for detailed instructions.

4. Can sea moss be consumed raw?

While it is possible to consume sea moss raw, it is recommended to soak and rinse it before consumption to ensure it is clean and free of possible contaminants.

5. Can sea moss be used in cooking?

Yes, sea moss can be used in cooking. It can be added to a variety of recipes and foods. Please check out the recipes chapter for ideas.

6. Are there any side effects of consuming sea moss?

While sea moss is generally safe for most people, some individuals might experience gut issues, allergic reactions, or adverse interactions with medications. Consult a healthcare professional before use.

7. Can sea moss be used as a skincare ingredient?

Yes, sea moss is commonly used in skincare products due to its potential benefits for the skin. Sea moss gel is also used directly to the face as a part of a skin care routine.

8. How do I use sea moss as a face mask?

Using your hands, apply sea moss gel evenly to your face. Allow the gel to dry on your skin. This usually takes about 15 minutes.

Once the gel has completely dried on the skin, rinse all the gel off your face with water and pat face dry.

9. Where can I buy sea moss?

Sea moss can be purchased from health food stores, specialty online retailers, or wholesale directly from suppliers. It is important to source sea moss from reputable sellers.

10. How should sea moss be stored?

Dried sea moss should be stored in a cool, dry place, away from moisture and direct sunlight.

Sea moss gel should be stored in an airtight sealed container. Sea moss gel must be refrigerated.

11. How long can sea moss gel be stored in the refrigerator?

Sea moss gel can be stored for two to three weeks. If you see white moldy bubbles, or particles forming on top of the sea moss gel, it has "expired." Do not consume.

12. Can sea moss be used during pregnancy or breastfeeding?

Pregnant or breastfeeding individuals should consult with their healthcare providers before incorporating sea moss or any new supplements into their diet.

Chapter 11

Other Resources

One of my main goals as an author, coach, and social media influencer is to help more than 100,000 people improve their health and weight. I know this is a lofty goal for just one person. But I'm up to the challenge! I have authored and published numerous resources to assist in plant-based nutritional knowledge, meal planning, fitness programming, and habit development. Please take advantage of these resources.

If you are already thinking about other ways to improve your health in addition to adding sea moss to your diet, my first book, "How to Eat Plant-Based Like a Boss," which is available on Amazon, is a great resource.

Here is the link for the paperback copy: https://amzn.to/2OpjsGE

Here is the link for the e-book: https://amzn.to/2txrTIE

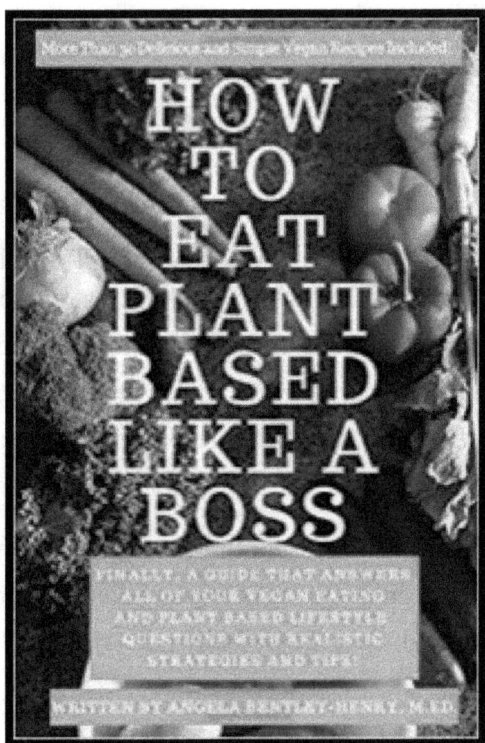

More Than 30 Delicious and Simple Vegan Recipes Included!

HOW TO EAT PLANT BASED LIKE A BOSS

FINALLY, A GUIDE THAT ANSWERS
ALL OF YOUR VEGAN EATING
AND PLANT BASED LIFESTYLE
QUESTIONS WITH REALISTIC
STRATEGIES AND TIPS!

WRITTEN BY ANGELA BENTLEY-HENRY, M.ED.

If you are looking for a great way to plan out your goals and keep track of your nutrition and workouts, here are some links to some great planners, logbooks, and journals:

Level Up Your Habits: Fitness, Nutrition, and Weight Tracker: Planner, Log, and Calendar

Here is the link https://amzn.to/39f3ve1

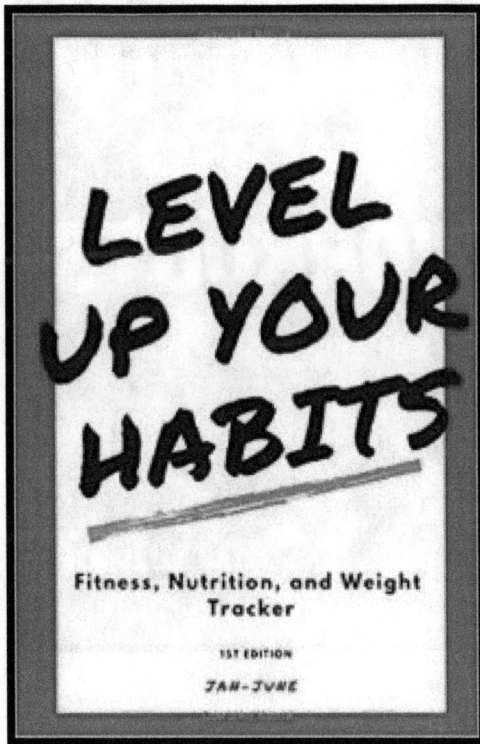

Level Up Your Workouts: Fitness Journal

Here is the link https://amzn.to/3AeKckG

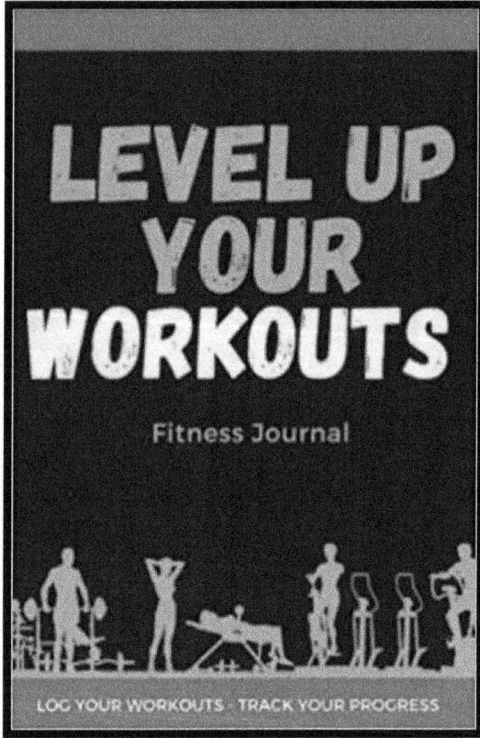

Level Up Your Nutrition: Food Journal and Meal Planner

Here is the link https://amzn.to/3MSKN2Z

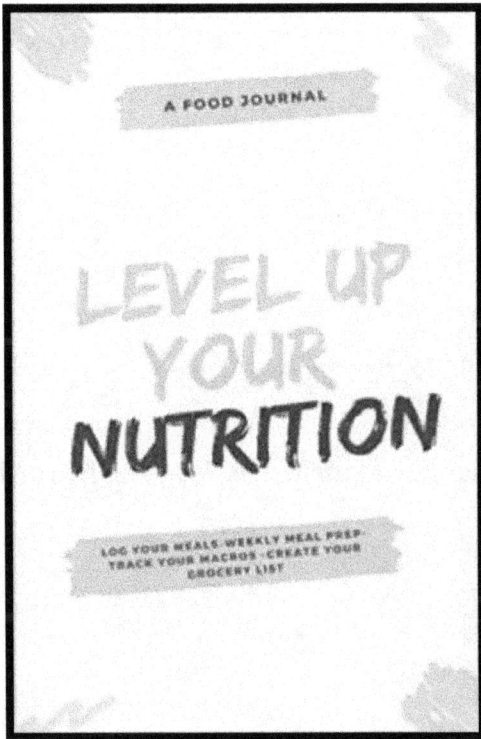

Be sure to keep in contact with me. I would love to hear about your successes and experiences along your health journey.

You can email me at letshealth@yahoo.com. You can message me on all social media platforms (Instagram, Facebook, and Tik Tok).

All resources, both published and digital downloads can be found at https://letshealth.biz/

If you share your journey and results on social media, please tag me @letshealthwithange and use the hashtag #LETSHEALTH

Now, go enjoy some sea moss and LETS Health!

About the Author

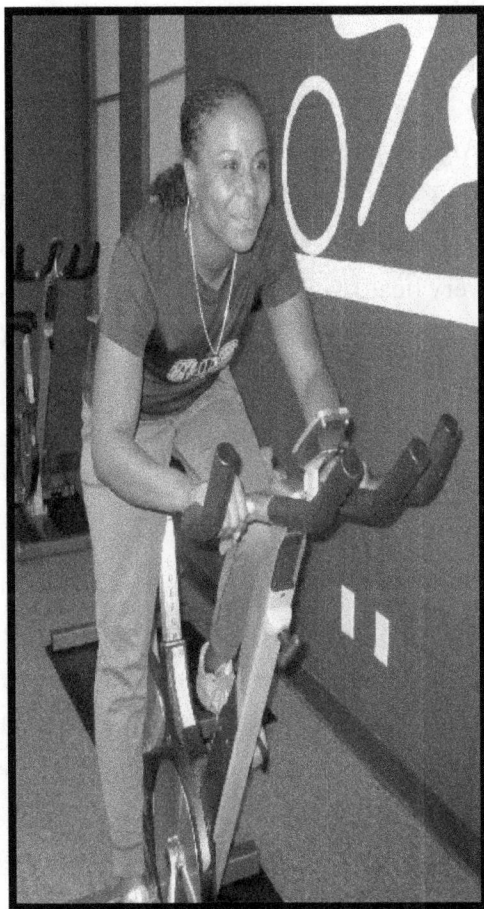

Educating and inspiring others to eat plant-based and live healthy and fit lifestyles is truly Angela's passion. Seeing others benefit from plant-based eating combined with physical activity is a personal mission that she has taken on since the death of her grandmother. Angela watched her grandmother fight a 20-year battle with diabetes (which led to strokes, feeding tubes, being wheelchair-bound, and needing a pacemaker). Before her grandmother's death, Angela did not know that there was a way to battle diabetes, hypertension, and other lifestyle diseases. She now believes in the power of plants. Her life has been the proof.

Angela grew up in a small town where healthy options weren't always available. She was very active throughout her childhood and teenage years. Angela played sports in school and was a standout basketball player. After college, she even had the opportunity to play semiprofessional basketball. Because of her active lifestyle, Angela appeared to be very healthy. She did not have any bodyweight issues and, thus, saw no reason to change the way she ate (which wasn't very plant-based). However, over time, those unhealthy eating habits caught up with her. In 2015 (the same year her grandmother passed away), Angela was diagnosed with pre-diabetes and was severely overweight.

She truly understands the desire a person has to live healthily while enjoying the foods they are eating. Loving the food she is eating, and recreating those foods in delicious and creative ways, has always been fun and important to her. Throughout her childhood and teenage years, Angela spent most weeknights and weekends experimenting with recipes in the kitchen with her mom and watching the Food Network. This same pleasure of cooking continues throughout her plant-based journey. Sharing delicious recipes with others brings her joy.

Plant-based eating is the reason why Angela has lost over 50 pounds and reversed her pre-diabetes. It is also how she is living a healthier, higher-quality life. By sharing the benefits of plant-based eating with others, as well as providing tips and suggestions for navigating the day-to-day experiences of eating plant-based, she wishes to improve the quality of life for many.

Angela truly believes that plants provide her with the fuel she needs to engage in activities she loves, like playing basketball, staying busy with her daughters, jumping rope, and working out. Angela hopes to inspire others to fuel their lives with plants as well.

Degrees:

- Master of Science in Education – Nova Southeastern University
- Graduate Certificate Nutrition (In Progress) -- Liberty University
- Bachelor of Science – University of Central Florida

Certifications:

- Plant-based Cooking – Rouxbe, Forks Over Knives
- Health Education – Florida Department of Education
- Physical Education – Florida Department of Education
- Weight Management Specialist – The National Council for Certified Personal Trainers
- Punk Rope Jump Rope Instructor – Punk Rope, Inc.

Professional:

- Physical Education and Health Teacher
- Track and Field Coach
- Brevard Public School, Healthy Liaison (School Based)
- Supplements Provider (Sea Moss, Herbal Tea)
- Life Insurance and Annuity Agent (Florida certified)

Publications and Resources:

- Author, "How to Eat Plant-based Like A Boss"
- Author, "Level Up Your Habits: Fitness, Nutrition, and Weight Tracker: Planner, Log, and Calendar"
- Author, "Level Up Your Workouts: Fitness Journal"
- Author, "Level Up your Nutrition: Food Log"
- Author, "3 Day Raw Cleanse Guide" (Digital Download)
- Author, "7 Day Plant Powered Challenge Guide" (Digital Download)

All these resources can be found at https://letshealth.biz/

Reference List

- https://medlineplus.gov/definitions/mineralsdefinitions.html
- https://www.medicinenet.com/13_essential_minerals/article.htm
- https://vegnews.com/vegan-guides/sea-moss-benefits
- https://en.wikipedia.org/wiki/Mastocarpus_stellatus
- https://agri.ohio.gov/divisions/food-safety/resources/sea-moss#:~:text=Chondrus%20Crispus%20(commonly%20referred%20to,moss%20used%20in%20food%20production.